Diabetic Chronicles

Life Stories of Diabetes Warriors

Tahar Das

Contents

Introduction

In a world where life's unpredictability can often throw us unexpected challenges, there exists a group of remarkable individuals whose stories stand as testaments to the extraordinary strength of the human spirit. Welcome to "Diabetic Chronicles: Life Stories of Diabetes Warriors." Within the pages of this book, you will embark on a journey into the lives of those who have faced the unrelenting trials and tribulations of living with diabetes.

Each story is a unique portal into a world where courage, resilience, and determination are not just words but a way of life. From the gripping account of a harrowing night in Kowloon where zombies and low blood sugar collide, to the heartwarming saga of a parent juggling student loans, type 1 diabetes, two kids, and a life spread across three states, the stories you are about to encounter will inspire and move you.

Prepare to be taken on a rollercoaster ride through the highs and lows of living with diabetes. In "Diabetes: A Date Night's Unexpected Turn," you will witness the power of love in the face of adversity. "T1D & Low Self-esteem" explores the inner battles that many warriors of this condition face, and "Living with Diabetes Is Difficult" delves into the daily struggles that are rarely seen but deeply felt.

But it's not all about hardship; you'll also share in moments of laughter and triumph. Discover the unexpected joys in "Diabetes: Fun Moments" and hear stories of transformation where diabetes became "The Best Thing That Happened" to some. From positive pregnancy experiences to achieving Keto success, and even running to beat diabetes, these chronicles are as diverse as the individuals behind them.

As we turn the pages of this collective narrative, you'll meet those who have carried the weight of type 1 diabetes since their teenage years and others who have embraced its presence as "A kind of nice T1D." You'll hear about the miraculous postpartum journeys and the incredible tales of survival, like escaping Preeclampsia's grasp.

With each story, you'll walk in the shoes of warriors who have faced their fears and fought against adversity. Through their experiences, you'll find inspiration, hope, and a profound understanding of what it means to be a diabetes warrior. "Diabetic Chronicles" invites you to join this community of extraordinary individuals and explore the intricate tapestry of their lives.

Get ready to be moved, enlightened, and inspired as you delve into the captivating narratives of these remarkable individuals who have turned the challenges of diabetes into a testament of their indomitable spirit. These are the stories of warriors who refused to let diabetes define them; instead, they became the authors of their own empowering chronicles.

Nightmare in Kowloon: Zombies and Low Blood Sugar

During my week-long layover in Hong Kong for visa renewal in December 2012, I embarked on a memorable adventure. After a four-day trek along the enchanting Maclehose path in the New Territories of Northern Hong Kong, I returned to Kowloon to celebrate the upcoming New Year with friends. The whole experience left me covered in dirt and pricker bush scratches, and I was in desperate need of a shower, a shave, and some relaxation.

When I find myself in Hong Kong without the luxury of a friend's couch to crash on, my go-to budget accommodation is the ten-dollar-a-night beds in Chung King Mansion, a somewhat rundown skyscraper situated in the heart of Kowloon. This place has always fascinated me because it's a melting pot of cultures—a haven for newcomers to the city. The first few floors boast a variety of shops and restaurants where you can find everything from pirated Bollywood DVDs to delectable Pakistani omelets. As you ascend the building, you'll discover affordable guest houses that cater to both short-term and long-term guests.

Back in the 1980s, Chung King Mansion was notorious for its lawlessness, a place where even the police feared to tread. It was a world of its own, where gangs, drugs, prostitution, delicious food, and the occasional crime thrived. Over the years, it has cleaned up its act, but it still retains a unique charm. To me, it's the perfect place to be an anonymous traveler.

So, there I was, on a sunny afternoon of December 31, 2012, planning to attend my fiddle teacher's performance at an Irish bar that evening and then celebrate the New Year with a friend. Finding an affordable place to crash was on my to-do list, and Chung King Mansion seemed like the perfect choice.

Now, if you're familiar with the process of finding a bed in Chung King, you'll know it's not always straightforward. You climb the stairs to the upper floors and knock on the doors of guest houses, attempting to communicate in Cantonese as best as you can. It often takes several tries before you find a bed, especially on a busy night like New Year's Eve.

Eventually, I managed to secure a bunk bed on the eighteenth floor, sharing the room with three other travelers. The room had a distinct aroma, a mixture of socks and a faint, stale scent of vomit. Two of the beds were a mess, strewn with laundry and the occasional toothbrush, while the third bed was occupied by an elderly, bearded man who seemed to be in deep slumber, almost like a pharaoh in a sarcophagus.

I couldn't help but watch him, intrigued by the deep wrinkles etched into his weathered face. However, something seemed off—his chest didn't rise and fall as it should. Was he possibly… dead? I gently placed my hand in front of his nostrils, but there was no perceptible breath. The situation was strange, but I wasn't sure how to handle it. After all, I wasn't well-versed in the etiquette of dealing with deceased roommates. I decided to check on him later when I returned from my evening plans.

But first, I needed a refreshing shower to wash away the dirt and grime accumulated from my recent hike. Afterward, I ventured out for a night of Irish tunes, potato wedges, and merry strangers singing "Wagon Wheel." Later, I met a friend at a rooftop bar in Causeway Bay, indulging in sweet herbed martinis and enjoying the New Year's fireworks over the harbor.

I was well-prepared for the night ahead, anticipating fluctuating blood sugar levels due to the celebrations. I estimated my carb intake on the higher side, keeping a roll of Mentos in my jacket, just in case. Sugar worries were the least of my concerns; I was here to have a fantastic time.

At around 2 in the morning, in a slightly tipsy state, I returned to Chung King Mansion, only to notice that the elderly man in my room hadn't moved at all. I checked my blood sugar levels—perfectly stable at 100—and drifted into a peaceful slumber, ringing in the new year with style.

My dreams that night were filled with a surreal scenario—a zombie apocalypse. It was one of those lucid dreams where I wasn't a spectator but an active participant, navigating through a world overrun by fast-moving zombies. As I ventured out into the city the previous night, it had been bustling with people, but now, it seemed like the majority had been transformed into zombies, and no one was even aware of it.

I awoke at 5 am with a strong belief that this nightmarish narrative was real. If I had taken the time to check my blood sugar, I would have found it dangerously low, likely around 40-50. My legs felt weak, and my lips tingled, either from the low sugar or the alcohol wearing off, or perhaps a combination of both.

With no time to waste, I realized that I needed to act quickly. Were there really zombies? I wasn't sure, but caution was paramount. Chung King Mansion, one of the most densely populated places on Earth, could become a tinderbox for a zombie outbreak. I decided to proceed cautiously.

Silently, I descended from my upper bunk, taking care not to wake the elderly man or the other two roommates I hadn't yet met. I slipped out of the room, cautiously peering around the corner. It was 5 am on New Year's Day, and the place was eerily quiet. I needed to get down from the eighteenth floor without drawing attention.

The elevators in Chung King Mansion were notoriously slow, and their arrival was accompanied by a distinctive ding. Suddenly, I spotted a figure out of the corner of my eye—a cleaning woman pushing a mop and bucket. She appeared normal but could turn into a threat in an instant if she noticed me. I pressed my body against a door jamb, keeping a close eye on her every move.

She eventually turned away, providing me with an opportunity to make a break for it. I rushed barefoot down eighteen flights of stairs, stopping on the eighth floor to listen for any signs of pursuit. Thankfully, it was silent. My heart raced, and I was acutely aware of the fragile line between life and death that I was tiptoeing on. Was this how it would all end? Not if I had any say in it.

As I continued my descent, I noticed something unusual—the lower stairwell, typically bustling with loiterers and drunks, was deserted. The walls were stained with red betel nut spit, but the fresh red splatters seemed out of place. Could it be just betel juice, or was something more sinister at play?

I silently sprinted down the remaining stairs, ensuring that each step was taken with utmost care to avoid making any noise. Emerging from the door into the back alley behind Chung King Mansion, I felt the cool winter air envelop me, a mix of seawater, stale cigarette smoke, masala, cheap incense, and steamed rice.

I navigated the narrow alleyways, making my way toward Nathan Road, the bustling heart of Kowloon, which was typically teeming with people at all hours. However, on this day, it resembled a ghost town. There were no cars, no taxis, no double-decker buses, and no street vendors offering their wares. The city had transformed into a lifeless, empty shell.

As I continued north along Nathan Road, I couldn't help but wonder if the authorities were aware of the zombie situation. Did they even have a plan for a zombie apocalypse? I knew my best chance of survival lay in heading for the hills to the north.

Going south toward Hong Kong Harbor would only lead to entrapment.

I veered into the narrow alleyways of Tsim Sha Tsui, Jordan, and Yau Ma Tei, staying hidden from the main road. After covering a few miles, I stumbled upon a payphone mounted on a wall. This could be my chance to alert the authorities, but I had never called the Hong Kong police before. Would they understand my imperfect Cantonese? What was the word for "zombie"?

After a few minutes of inner debate, I picked up the receiver, hoping the operator would speak English and that I could make them understand the gravity of the situation.

"Hello? Yes, hello. I'm calling to tell you about a zombie outbreak in Hong Kong.

…

Yes, yes, zombies. The city is overrun with them.

….

My name? Sure (who has time for names now? They're missing the point. I give a pseudonym, just in case)

…

Yes, most people are zombies. I don't know how it happened.

…

Yes, I'm ok, for now. They haven't found me yet.

Who are they? The zombies, of course. Like I've been trying to tell you!"

As I struggled to convey the urgency of the situation, I realized that my low blood sugar was wreaking havoc on my ability to articulate my thoughts. Lows had always scrambled the link between my thoughts and words. It was frustrating, but I had to make the operator understand.

...

Have you ever had one of those moments where your whole mind was set on one reality suddenly dissolved around you? You realize that one or all of your core assumptions are wrong, and everything you built on that foundation is a pile of rubble?

I had never experienced this before my diabetes diagnosis and the intense waking dreams that came with low blood sugar. As I spoke to the operator, the cracks in my reality began to widen. Why wasn't I wearing any shoes? How did I know my life was in danger? Had I truly run for my life from a cleaning lady?

The operator on the phone continued to ask if I was okay.

"My mistake. There are no zombies. Everything's fine. (Like a Mafia victim telling the cops that they fell down the stairs)

...

Yes, sorry, I was mistaken. I shouldn't have called you."

I hung up the phone, embarrassed by my erroneous call. My mind cleared as the effects of low blood sugar waned. It was now six hours into the first day of 2013. I was cold, shoeless, and two miles away from my bed. The streets were deserted because of the holiday, and most people were nursing their hangovers. I had no wallet or subway card, so I had no choice but to embark on the long walk back.

Upon returning to Chung King Mansion, I took the elevator back up to the eighteenth floor. I had left in a hurry and without my keys, so I had to knock on the grated door for entry. The cleaning lady let me in, giving me a suspicious look. I considered offering her an explanation but decided against it. I muttered a quiet "thank you" and retreated to my room.

The elderly man still lay in his bed, unmoving, for the past eighteen hours. While he might not have been the best roommate, at least I knew he wasn't a zombie. I climbed into my bunk, finally able to get some much-needed sleep.

And so, my New Year's adventure in the heart of Kowloon took a surreal turn, a mix of dreamlike encounters, imaginary zombies, and the reality of life with diabetes. As I drifted off to sleep, I couldn't help but wonder what other surprises the city had in store for me in the days to come.

Student Loans, T1D, Two Kids, and a Saga Across Three States

Inception (Post Undergrad Years) - The Origin Story (23M/21F)

Our journey began in our final year of undergrad, where we both majored in Molecular Biology. Our paths converged, and we fell in love. I had initially started as an Aerospace Engineering major, but that's a story for another time.

My wife decided to pursue medicine initially, but after shadowing doctors and considering the mounting debt, she opted for a medical profession with more flexibility in specialties. This decision steered her away from med school, and we both entered the workforce in the fall of 2010.

I began my career as a research embryologist, while my wife worked towards her MCAT. I started with around $23k in student loan debt from undergrad, earning $15/hour. To make the most of it, I stayed on my parent's medical insurance, essentially adding an extra dollar to my hourly wage.

We were offered a 401k plan with no matching, and I initially didn't contribute. I did manage to work some overtime, up to

1.5 hours per week, whenever possible. At this point, my net worth was a bleak -$23k.

My wife landed a research assistant job at a State University lab, making $31k. This position included a rare automatic contribution to a pension plan, with payouts beginning at age 65 based on years of service. She had taken enough college-level courses in high school to complete her bachelor's in just three years, avoiding student loans. Her net worth was around $8k, thanks to savings accumulated over the years.

We moved in together, splitting expenses 50/50. I used my leftover money after monthly bills to chip away at my student loans, although I foolishly didn't maintain an emergency fund. My wife and I had our share of debates about this financial choice, but eventually, I established a $500 safety net.

We both excelled in our jobs, and two years in, I managed to increase my pay to $17/hour, still benefiting from the extra dollar by opting out of health insurance. I had reduced my student loan balance to about $10k but hadn't started contributing to retirement or saving much.

My wife, however, was itching to pursue a career in medicine. She considered Physician Assistant (PA) school for its specialization flexibility over traditional med school. To gain the necessary patient hours, she transitioned to a role as a Clinical Research Coordinator at the University. This came with a pay increase to $41k and continued pension plan contributions.

As we got engaged, my wife was accepted into PA school in another state, prompting me to leave my job and move with her. It seemed like a good opportunity for me to pursue further education. I had been taking online courses in statistics and programming, and I saw bioinformatics as a way to blend biology and computer science.

Thankfully, I found a remote master's program that aligned with my goals, starting simultaneously with my wife's PA school journey. As we left our jobs, our combined net worth was around $0, with my $10k in undergrad loans still outstanding and my wife's $10k in savings.

Back to School and the Weight of Debt (26M/24F)

My master's program spanned 24 months, while my wife's PA program took 27. Her program restricted outside employment to avoid interfering with rotations and coursework. We both refrained from working during our grad school years, further increasing our reliance on loans.

I am a Type I Diabetic, and I needed comprehensive insurance coverage. The ACA's passage meant I couldn't be denied due to my preexisting condition. I purchased an insurance plan that covered my diabetes care but came with premiums and co-insurance, all funded through our student loans.

By the end of our educational journey, we had accumulated $250k in student loans, including interest. I had one internship that paid $6k, but other than that, our lives were fully financed by loans. Most of it went to tuition, medical expenses, and rent, though we allowed ourselves some occasional indulgences like dining out, alcohol, and entertainment. We also managed to keep our wedding costs under $5k.

Graduation, Career Kickoff, Parenthood, and Health Challenges (28M/26F)

Following graduation, I landed a job offer from my internship, and we moved to yet another state. I started with a salary of $72k, boasting a generous benefits package that included a 9% 401K match, an HSA with a $2,000 automatic employer contribution, and health and dental insurance.

My wife followed a few months later, securing a position as a PA in a rheumatology practice. Her initial role was contract-to-hire, paying $40/hour without retirement benefits but including medical coverage, which she declined as we both used my work plan.

With a combined net worth of approximately -$240k, we dove headfirst into our new careers. We experienced rapid advancements and substantial raises, averaging an 8% increase in pay per year as a couple. My wife's contract turned into a full-time job, with her salary increasing to $100k and a 4% retirement match if she contributed 6% of her base salary.

Our growing interest in personal finance led us to meticulously track our expenses, first with Mint and later with YNAB. We made sure to contribute enough to secure our retirement match, allocating the rest towards chipping away at our student loans.

Working in a high-cost-of-living area, we initially opted for an older apartment complex. Three years ago, we moved to a townhouse, paying $2,000 per month for a 3/2.5 unit close to work, eliminating the need for a long commute.

As we witnessed the progress on our student loans, our enthusiasm for personal finance grew. We discovered the concept of financial independence, which had to wait while we prioritized paying off our loans. We only considered ourselves financially free once our remaining loans carried an interest rate of less than 4.5%, totaling around $30k.

After six months of working, our net worth improved to -$200k, and it dropped to -$150k after a year. We managed to increase our net worth by paying off student loans at a pace of approximately $100k per year for nearly five years.

In August 2018, as our first child was born, we hit a net worth of $0. Just before our child's birth, I underwent a kidney removal surgery due to a genetic condition that caused it to fill with fluid, disrupting its function. Fortunately, our maximum medical expenses were covered by insurance, as we had already hit our out-of-pocket maximum due to my diabetes.

The Present Day (33M/31F)

We celebrated the payoff of our student loans and reached a net worth of $150k in January of 2020. Our second child was born in March, just before the pandemic took hold.

Luckily, we both retained our jobs and salaries during the pandemic, allowing us to reach a net worth of $250k this month. My parents, who had retired a few years earlier, and my mother, who was forced into retirement by the pandemic, have kindly agreed to watch our children while we work.

We've transitioned from aggressively paying off debt to focusing on saving for retirement, giving us a taste of financial freedom. Our journey has been marked by hard work, some fortunate circumstances, and a radical shift in our lives that has significantly benefited us.

I'm trying to repair the damage

In the autumn of 1993, just a couple of months before my sixth birthday, my world began to change. I had been steadily losing weight, feeling perpetually tired, and battling persistent illness for several months. Concerned, my family decided to take me to a nearby children's hospital, where I would embark on a week-long journey of treatment and education.

At that tender age, I was overwhelmed by fear and confusion, while my parents grappled with their own heartache. My dad's youngest brother had been diagnosed with type 1 diabetes almost two decades earlier, and my mom had several relatives dealing with type 2 diabetes. It was a family issue we were all too familiar with.

In those days, insulin pens were unheard of, and pumps were reserved for rare and extreme cases, at least in central Iowa. My daily routine involved injections of Regular and NPH insulin to manage my blood sugar levels.

Over the ensuing years, I faced various challenges at school while witnessing remarkable advancements in insulin technology. The glucometers I used evolved in terms of speed, accuracy, and the amount of blood required for testing.

My struggle with being different from my peers led me down a perilous path. I began indulging in foods from the "restricted list" – the foods my doctor and parents had prohibited to help control my blood sugar levels. Eventually, I transitioned from Regular insulin to the then-new Humalog.

In fifth grade, as puberty began to exert its influence, I experienced my first episode of Diabetic Ketoacidosis (DKA) and found myself in the ICU. After a subsequent DKA scare, I was switched to the newer Novolog. Despite these adjustments, I continued to battle control issues and ended up spending several weekends each year receiving treatment for ketoacidosis.

It wasn't until the summer before 8th grade, after enduring several unpleasant encounters with my school nurse regarding my treatment, that I finally agreed to try an insulin pump – the MiniMed 530, exclusively using Novolog. Fortunately, my weekends in the ICU became a thing of the past.

The initial month with the pump was marked by daily candy bar indulgences, as I tried to make up for the years I'd gone without enjoying real candy.

High school came and went, with occasional explanations of my diabetes and treatment needed for faculty and staff. Before graduating, I transitioned to the MiniMed Paradigm.

Upon entering college, I embarked on a decade-long journey of neglecting my blood sugar levels and dietary choices. I felt fine, but my already shaky control was rapidly deteriorating. The day after I graduated, I lost my insurance coverage through my dad.

Employment opportunities with insurance were scarce, forcing me to ration my diabetes supplies. With my finances stretched thin, even affording food became a challenge.

Finally, around the age of 27, I found a stable job with insurance coverage and rekindled my commitment to self-care.

In the years that followed, I managed to bring my A1c levels down from a concerning 11.6 to a more manageable 6.9. Along the way, I received a diagnosis of macular edema as a result of diabetic eye disease and began treatment for it. Currently, I rely on the MiniMed 770 as I strive to undo the damage caused during my tumultuous teenage and early adult years.

As I approach nearly three decades of living with diabetes, I've witnessed numerous advancements in diabetes treatment and care. The journey has been far from easy, but it has shaped me into the resilient individual I am today.

Diabetes: A Date Night's Unexpected Turn

Last night, my diabetes threw me a curveball and presented me with an unexpected opportunity to see just how cool someone could be. Turns out, they're pretty darn cool, and I'm definitely smitten!

It was our third date, and we decided to meet at a Thai restaurant for dinner. Like many of you, Thai cuisine ranks high on my list of favorites, but it can be quite challenging to calculate insulin dosages for. I mentally prepped myself to keep an eye on my blood sugar numbers without making it seem weird or awkward.

As I headed out for our date, I noticed I had about eight units left in my insulin pump. I knew that after indulging in a delicious Thai meal, I'd need to change everything out. Wasting even a single unit of insulin wasn't an option, so I made the choice not to switch things up before our date.

Over dinner, I decided to broach the topic of my diabetes. It was only our third date, and we were still in the process of discovering each other's quirks and potential deal breakers.

Diabetes had the potential to be one of those deal breakers, so I thought it best to bring it up relatively early in our relationship.

I explained the delicate balance I have to maintain daily—a constant equation involving insulin, food, and exercise. I kept it simple, avoiding getting bogged down in the nitty-gritty details. I shared why I'm hyper-aware of physical activity and what I eat, and how I meticulously plan every aspect of my life, only to have those plans occasionally thwarted by diabetes.

I touched upon potential complications but reassured them that my risk was relatively low. To my relief, the conversation flowed smoothly, and it seemed like diabetes wasn't a deal breaker after all. Phew!

After dinner, I mentioned that I needed to quickly change my insulin pump before we headed to a bar for an after-dinner drink. I was a tad self-conscious about doing this, but, hey, welcome to my life—there's no time like the present to find out if this is a deal breaker or not.

So, I began the process of filling the reservoir, removing the old set, and preparing to replace the reservoir and set. But here's where it took an unexpected turn—I realized I'd forgotten to pack a new set in my bag! Ugh! I grabbed the reservoir and the two needle components but left the infusion set behind. (By the way, Tandem's recent change of separating the needle pieces into two separate packages threw me off twice this week because it increased the number of pieces from 3 to 4.)

I panicked and emptied the contents of my bag onto the car seat, but there was no sign of the missing infusion set. A string of choice words crossed my mind. I was 15 minutes away from home, and there was no way I could do anything else but head home. After all, I had just devoured a Thai feast!

I took a deep breath and looked at my date. They could already sense that something was amiss. I explained that I had to go home urgently because I was missing a crucial piece of my insulin pump and couldn't afford to be disconnected for long. Amazingly, they calmly and without any complaints told me it was okay. They offered to follow me home, and we'd figure things out from there. So, that's exactly what we did.

In the end, my blood sugar levels peaked at 275 that night, and I unintentionally gave them a hands-on lesson in how diabetes can throw a wrench into even the best-laid plans. Yet, through it all, I had the privilege of witnessing their kindness and understanding. I'm pretty confident there'll be more dates in our future (once I'm back in town next month, for different reasons).

Ah, the adventures of dating with diabetes—it's always an interesting ride!

T1D & Low self-esteem

I was diagnosed with Type 1 diabetes when I was just 4 years old. Fast forward to today, I'm 25 years old, managing my condition with FSL 2, Fiasp, and Lantus from pens, and I've come a long way.

My last A1c reading was 5.7, but I've had my fair share of hypos. Fortunately, that has improved since my last lab test, and my A1c hasn't crossed the 6.6 mark for over four years now.

My memories from that initial hospital stay at the age of 4 are somewhat hazy, but one thing I remember vividly is the doctor who treated me there. He eventually became my endocrinologist for a few years, and honestly, I couldn't stand the guy. Needles and blood draws were his specialty, and I felt like a human pincushion.

Managing diabetes was a tough journey for me, especially up until around age 15. I was overweight, struggled immensely with blood glucose control, and my self-esteem was at an all-time low.

However, things took a turn during my 15th year on this planet when I decided to start a diet. It was nothing fancy, just calorie counting and long walks at first. Eventually, I summoned the courage to step into a gym. I went from 90kg to just under 60kg, and my blood glucose management started to improve.

Yes, there were moments when I'd see that scale tip back to 90kg, but this time it was different. I had traded fat for muscle, and that positively impacted my blood glucose control. If you're curious, look up the Warburg effect. It's rooted in cancer research but seems to have implications for muscle hypertrophy as well. Essentially, growing cells switch up their metabolism to gobble up more carbs, using that carbon for growth. While still somewhat speculative, the evidence seems to be mounting.

That's why I affectionately refer to my quads as my "Anti-diabetes" engine. After a heavy session of resistance exercises like barbell squats, my insulin needs drop by roughly a third. I firmly believe in the power of heavy resistance training for people with Type 1 diabetes. But enough about that; let's move on.

Low self-esteem, as I mentioned earlier, was something I battled with. However, it's not tied to my diabetes, at least I hope not. Over the years, I've learned not to care about people's reactions to my T1-related behaviors. I'll inject my insulin in the middle of a bustling mall if that's what my body needs. No more rushing to bathrooms just to hide what I need to do to keep my metabolism ticking. I've embraced the "take it or leave it" attitude when it comes to my condition, and it's made all the difference.

Living with Diabetes Is Difficult

I received my Type 1 diabetes diagnosis at the age of 26, and now, at 30, I've come quite a long way. When I was first diagnosed, my A1c was a daunting ten, but through dedication and perseverance, I've managed to bring it down to a more manageable 7.

Diabetes has a familial connection in my case, as my father has Type 1, and my mother is a nurse. It was actually a conversation with my mother that led to my diagnosis. I mentioned having persistent mouth sores that just wouldn't go away. She promptly tested my blood sugar, and the result was shocking— my levels were in the 400s. Thankfully, we caught it early.

For the initial few months, I was misdiagnosed as having Type 2 diabetes by my general doctor. He prescribed pills that seemed to work, probably because I was still producing some insulin at the time. However, I decided to consult a specialist who conducted more comprehensive blood work, leading to a corrected diagnosis of Type 1. I was then switched to injections, which became a daily routine.

Within a year, my body stopped producing insulin altogether, and I found myself relying on insulin pens. Two years ago, I made another transition, this time to an insulin pump and continuous glucose monitor (CGM), which has significantly improved my diabetes management.

Juggling a busy job often made it challenging for me to find the time to remember to administer insulin injections, which is why the switch to an insulin pump and CGM has been a game-changer. Nevertheless, I'm aware that I still have work to do to further improve my A1c.

One of the biggest hurdles I've faced in my journey has been navigating the intricacies of insurance and the financial burden of managing my condition. It's disheartening to realize that I must spend thousands of dollars each year to maintain my health and simply stay alive.

Being diagnosed with Type 1 diabetes later in life presented its own set of challenges. I had already settled into my career and established a certain lifestyle, which made it harder to adapt. But as they say, it is what it is. Life can be tough, but I'm determined to face these challenges head-on and continue to work towards better health and well-being.

I'm Going Strong Now

I've been living with diabetes for a remarkable 21 years now, and my journey has been nothing short of eventful. It all began with a week of relentless thirst and frequent trips to the bathroom, which culminated in an embarrassing incident in my classroom. My teacher's insensitivity during that moment left a lasting impression, but ultimately, my health took precedence.

Coincidentally, my younger brother had been diagnosed with Type 1 diabetes a year prior, so my parents recognized the telltale signs when they saw them in me. With a sense of urgency, I visited the doctor to get the confirmation I feared.

Now, let me share a bit about the state of our local hospital system. It had a reputation for being more concerned with profits than patients, and it had changed ownership multiple times due to malpractice and questionable practices. Unfortunately, my firsthand experience with this system was far from reassuring.

In the ER, my glucose levels were so off the charts that their equipment couldn't even read them. It was a grim indication of my condition. The doctor tasked with inserting an IV line made an alarming oversight, leaving the line open, causing blood to flow freely. I was in a state of distress, too ill to comprehend what was happening. It took a second visit from the doctor to rectify the situation, his cavalier attitude unnerving me.

Adding to the ordeal, another physician at the hospital attempted to misdiagnose me as a Type 2 diabetic, which I met with a defiant laugh and a one-finger salute as I walked out of the office. Yes, this all occurred in the United States, where our healthcare system is unfortunately notorious for its flaws, a fact well-known to many diabetics.

Refusing to subject myself to such inadequate care, I made the decision to seek healthcare in another state, where I found a doctor who was not only a healthcare professional but also a fellow Type 1 diabetic. His guidance and expertise were a godsend, helping me turn my diabetes management around.

Today, I'm thriving with a continuous glucose monitor (CGM) and an A1C of 7.1. I've managed to keep diabetic complications at bay through regular exercise, a mostly keto diet, and a healthy dose of hydration. I've even tackled mountain trail runs, proving that diabetes doesn't have to define my limitations.

However, my brother's journey has taken a different turn. His diabetes management has been challenging, leading to the loss of toes and teeth, and he's now at risk of full amputations. He's on the transplant list due to his health complications, which were exacerbated by unconventional treatments like using marijuana to manage his diabetes—an approach that, in his case, clearly didn't work as intended.

It Looked Like a Bullet Wound

Back in my college days, I was a die-hard punk fan (and still am). Whenever a great punk band came to town, you could bet I'd be there, ready to rock out. One memorable night, I headed to the House of Blues with a bunch of friends to catch NOFX in action.

We pre-gamed, got the party started, and during the concert, I enjoyed a couple of beers while soaking in the epic atmosphere of the mosh pit. By the time the show concluded, I was drenched in sweat, battered from the moshing, and slightly intoxicated. With my friends heading back to their dorms, I decided to make the trek up the hill to my campus residence.

As I trudged up that hill, my trusty Omnipod piped up with its beeping, indicating that it was time to change to a new pod since the three days were up. Now, in my inebriated state, that beep was grating on my nerves. I figured I could cancel the current pod, chuck it in a nearby trash can, and replace it with a fresh one once I got back to my room.

However, thanks to the hour I'd spent enthusiastically moshing and bumping into fellow concertgoers, the injection site had gotten rather bloody. When I removed the Omnipod and tossed it, I noticed I was bleeding quite profusely from the spot. The realization dawned on me when I felt my pocket grow damp. And to make matters more interesting, I was wearing a light-colored off-white shirt that would inevitably reveal any stains.

Faced with this situation and a lack of tissues or anything to clean up with, I resorted to pressing my T-shirt against the bleeding site. It was time for a quick solution, so I decided to make a pitstop at the residence office since it was closer than my dorm. My mission: grab some trusty paper towels.

As I walked into the office, the two RAs on duty that night happened to be inside, engaged in conversation. The sight of me, with my wet, reddish-stained shirt, startled them into silence. To their wide-eyed shock, it seemed as though I'd taken a bullet to the chest!

In my slightly slurred speech, I muttered that I needed to freshen up. In the well-lit office, I finally realized how soaked and crimson my shirt had become, and I couldn't help but chuckle at how much it resembled a gunshot wound. The RAs, still bewildered, exchanged incredulous glances. I paused for a moment, looked at them, and simply remarked, "I had a crazy night." No further explanation was needed. I grabbed my paper towels, headed to the bathroom, and walked out with a story to remember.

Diabetes: Fun Moments

I used to use Omnipod for a while to give it a test run and had left my meter for it to a family member. It was time to change it and suffice it to say that little motherf****r was beeping so loud at 3 AM that I was beside myself, especially given that my mother was asleep downstairs.

I did the only rational thing I knew to do, made a full sprint to the front door, and chucked that shit as far as I could; problem solved. Also, remember this happening another time, I believe again at night, and I got a pot of water, threw it in there, shut the lid, wrapped the pot in a towel, and buried it in the furthest possible closet from my bedroom. Those little shits were annoying when they beeped.

Also, even though this one might be perceived as more scary than funny, it's not what happened; it's how it happened. I was staying at my buddy's house when I was 11, and I remember going to bed with good blood sugar without considering that we had been running around ALL day.

So, I fell during the night. I woke up with my vision spinning and was on a mission to the fridge. I was so disoriented that I started shoveling ice cream out of the carton with my bare hands. Gross, I know, but I was in the process of dying. The worst part is that, unbeknownst to my friend's family, I just stuck it back in there and acted like nothing ever happened.

I used to date a girl who was diligent and caring about my diabetes and encouraged me to take better care of myself. This may be TMI, but suffice it to say we were rabbits when I suddenly lost my hard-on and was mortified.

It was funny that she wasn't even worried about it and was still supportive. After my 'juice break,' I went on to have killer sex, and we could laugh about it in the future. It just helped turn fear into fun.

Diabetes: The Best Thing That Happened to Me

As the summer of 2015 approached, I was immersed in my finals, which were just three weeks away. Suddenly, I fell ill with a severe flu that kept me bedridden for three days. Fearing the worst, I decided to visit a private doctor whom I had occasionally seen in the past.

My usual doctor was unavailable that day, so I agreed to see another physician at the clinic. After examining me, this doctor prescribed Amoxil Antibiotic for my illness. I began taking Amoxil, but after three days, I started to experience excruciating joint pain and an intense itch all over my body that kept getting worse. Concerned, I shared this with my parents.

My mother, after reviewing my list of allergies, recalled that I had G6PD and realized this could be related. My father promptly contacted our family doctor, who advised us to rush to the hospital. There, I received a cortisone injection to alleviate my symptoms and was allowed to return home. Although the itch subsided, the joint pain lingered.

A day later, still in discomfort, my parents and I rushed back to the hospital for another cortisone shot. After the second injection, the joint pain finally began to fade, allowing me to return to school the following day.

School ended, and the Holy Month of Ramadan began in our country. I was entering my second year of fasting during Ramadan and felt confident about it. However, as soon as Ramadan ended, my family decided to take a trip to London. Upon arriving, I collapsed onto my bed and woke up the next day with an urgent need to urinate. I rushed to the bathroom and emptied my bladder.

I didn't mention this to my family at the time, as it didn't seem like a significant concern. However, while we were at Harrods, I suddenly felt an overwhelming need to urinate again. I couldn't hold it in, and I realized I needed to return to our hotel room immediately. Once there, as I closed the bathroom door behind me, I was hit by a massive headache and drenched in sweat, despite the room being comfortably cool.

Although I was frightened by what was happening, I chose not to worry my family with my concerns. Throughout our 21-day stay in London, my personality underwent a dramatic transformation. I went from being a cheerful, carefree kid to someone who was moody, irritable, and prone to emotional outbursts.

Upon returning to our home country, I started attending a new school. Alongside my changing personality, I began experiencing sleepless nights, frequent urination, and an insatiable thirst. I eventually shared these symptoms with my parents, and we rushed to our family doctor.

The doctor questioned me about my daily water intake, which had increased to around 15-16 bottles daily from almost none previously. This drastic change alarmed me. However, the doctor attributed it to my growing body.

Over the next three months, my health continued to deteriorate. I struggled to stay awake at school, neglected my homework, consumed excessive amounts of water, and barely ate. I experienced tremors and excessive sweating.

During this time, I underwent a blood test at the doctor's request. Days after the test, I returned home with my friends, only to be abruptly called to the car by my mother, who appeared deeply concerned. I left my friends behind and headed to the emergency room with my mother.

As they tested my blood sugar levels, they found them alarmingly high at 400 mg/dL. An A1c test confirmed a reading of 9.1. At that moment, I had no comprehension of what this meant for my health, assuming my blood sugar levels were normal.

I spent the next three days in the hospital, where I received essential education on managing diabetes. I learned how to inject myself, the importance of carb counting, and the basics of self-care. It was September 29, 2015, when I was diagnosed.

Looking back, I've come to realize that being diagnosed with diabetes was one of the best things that happened to me. It forced me to see life from a different perspective and helped me understand how I could benefit from this diagnosis.

T1D: Positive Pregnancy & Birth Experience

As I embarked on this journey, I was understandably anxious, knowing that each pregnancy and delivery is unique. My hope is that my story can provide reassurance to women in a similar situation, as I was just like them nine months ago, hoping for a healthy and positive pregnancy experience.

I've been living with diabetes for 27 years, a long journey that began without a blood glucose meter during the first year or two, relying solely on color-changing test strips. Despite the challenges, I've been fortunate not to have obvious retinopathy or other complications. While my A1c levels were not always ideal, ranging between seven and 8 for many years, I was determined to improve them when I decided to pursue pregnancy.

My endocrinologist advised me to aim for A1c levels below seven and closer to 6 if possible. It didn't happen overnight, but after years of trying to conceive (ultimately discovering that male infertility, not type 1 diabetes, was the issue), I finally received a positive pregnancy test with an A1c around 6.

In addition to diabetes, I also manage celiac disease, MS, and Hashimoto's. Fortunately, none of these conditions had a negative impact on my pregnancy, and I maintained good overall health, even while continuing to run long distances and handle a demanding job.

Upon receiving the positive test, I became hyper-focused on my blood sugar levels, perhaps a bit too much. The stress of trying to achieve perfect control began to affect my mental health, even though my A1c results during pregnancy were impressive at 4.7, 4.7, and 4.8. Despite these excellent results, I still encountered occasional high spikes, particularly during the early and late stages of pregnancy, as well as frequent lows, with weeks 8-12 being particularly challenging and occasionally frightening. I want to emphasize that experiencing high spikes in the first few weeks of pregnancy does not mean your pregnancy is doomed.

I found several strategies helpful in managing my blood sugar levels. This included dosing insulin ahead of meals, starting with 30 minutes before eating (increasing to 60 minutes in the third trimester), opting for low glycemic index carbohydrates (such as chickpea flour pasta and pizza crust, almond flour desserts, although I did indulge in simple carbs during the first trimester), and maintaining a regular walking and hiking routine.

I saw an endocrinologist every month or two but largely managed my own care. I also followed the typical pregnancy schedule with my OB, including weekly non-stress tests (NSTs) starting at 35 weeks, and had appointments with a maternal-fetal medicine (MFM) doctor every two weeks from around 24 weeks onwards. The MFM doctor often took a more conservative approach, expressing concerns about possible placental vascular complications due to my long history of diabetes. In contrast, my OB remained positive, as the baby consistently measured around the 45th percentile in all scans.

Throughout my pregnancy, I heard that induction would likely occur between weeks 37 and 38. However, when those weeks arrived, my OB suggested aiming for delivery between weeks 39 and 40. Initially, this change scared me, and the MFM doctor was also cautious about it. However, we eventually scheduled an induction at 39+3 days, as the baby continued to appear healthy during scans and NSTs.

To my surprise, labor began on its own at 39+1 weeks, shortly after I had gone on a long hike, and my water broke. I experienced a remarkably typical labor, lasting just under 24 hours from when my water broke, and I delivered vaginally. Fortunately, there were no unusual delivery complications, and our baby girl arrived alert, weighing 7 pounds and 4 ounces, with normal blood sugar levels.

Remarkably, the hospital staff allowed me to manage my diabetes throughout the labor process, with my husband recording my blood sugar levels hourly for their records. I brought along plenty of juice boxes, although I didn't end up needing many. Surprisingly, I was also allowed to eat during most of the labor, even without an epidural.

Now, I'm a week postpartum, and my blood sugar levels have been behaving erratically. However, it's all worth it for my sweet little girl. I hope that in future (hopefully!) pregnancies, I can have a similar positive experience. Having reasonable control was essential in ensuring our baby was a suitable size for a vaginal delivery, and having an OB who didn't push for unnecessary interventions played a crucial role in shaping this positive experience.

A kind of nice T1D

I'm on my way to becoming a nurse through an accelerated year program for a BSN. I've been living with type 1 diabetes since 1989, so that's 28 years now. Thankfully, I haven't experienced any complications apart from slightly elevated blood pressure.

During my nursing program, I've been immersing myself in studying various disease processes like heart failure, myocardial infarctions, renal failure, and more. It's been a bit disheartening because diabetes mellitus always seems to be listed as "2-4 times more at risk" for these conditions. It's hard not to let that weigh on your mind, even though I've always thought that making it to 60 would be a significant achievement. I've been grateful for the good quality of life I've maintained.

However, my perspective took a positive turn when I started my clinical rotation. We had an elderly patient admitted who was an 83-year-old type 1 diabetic, diagnosed at the tender age of 6. It was incredible to hear about his journey, from the days of testing his blood sugar with urine and using boiled needles to where we are today with advanced diabetes management techniques.

Talking to him further, I learned that he had taken excellent care of himself over the years by monitoring his diet and maintaining a healthy lifestyle. Surprisingly, he still used injections for insulin delivery instead of pump therapy and had no knowledge of CGMs, which I introduced to him.

What truly inspired me was that despite being in stage 4 renal failure and undergoing dialysis, he was 83 years old and still living life to the fullest. He had undergone laser eye surgery to address some issues and had experienced some neuropathy, but aside from that, he had remarkably few complications.

This encounter with him reminded me that if you take care of yourself and manage your diabetes well, you can enjoy everyday life to the fullest extent possible. It was a lesson in resilience and determination that left a lasting impact on me.

T1D Keto Success with 20:4 IF & no exercise

I want to share my remarkable journey of transformation from September to March. I've had type 1 diabetes since I was 12, and now at 29, I've experienced quite a journey.

Before I delve into my story, it's essential to understand that living with type 1 diabetes can be financially challenging, especially in a place like the United States. I spend around $15,000 to $20,000 each year on everything I need to manage my diabetes. With time, I noticed that I was becoming increasingly insulin resistant, requiring nearly three times the amount of insulin I was initially prescribed.

This predicament led me to consider the ketogenic diet. Not only would it potentially alleviate insulin resistance, but it could also help reduce the financial burden of buying so much insulin.

September 1st - Part 1

My journey began on September 1st. It took about five days to enter ketosis. During the first two weeks, my weight dropped from 278 to 260, primarily due to shedding water weight. As the month progressed, I continued to lose weight, eventually reaching 247. What astounded me was that I had to reduce my daily insulin from 44 units to 24, as taking more risked sending my blood sugar plummeting.

Being a type 1 diabetic on keto requires careful balancing. I must take enough insulin to stay alive but avoid excess that might lower my blood sugar too much. If it drops too low, I have to consume carbs to raise it, potentially knocking me out of ketosis. Knowing I had an upcoming vacation where I would break keto, I adhered to the diet until my birthday on October 10th.

October 21st - Part 2

I recommenced my keto journey on October 21st, starting at 257 pounds after taking a week off for my vacation. Luckily, the ketogenic diet isn't too challenging for someone with type 1 diabetes. I was already well-versed in counting carbs and understood the intricacies of managing my blood sugar.

January 14th - Part 3

By January 14th, I had been on keto for three months and weighed 218 pounds. The holiday season had its challenges, but I managed to stay on track. What's even more astonishing, my eating disorder (ED) vanished, and my confidence skyrocketed. I hadn't needed to buy new clothes for a while because I could fit into my old ones and even garments I had bought but never returned. To top it off, I became more insulin-sensitive, now requiring only 20 units a day, down from 44 when I started.

March 24th - Part 4

My current weight sits at 198.6 pounds, and my goal is to dip below 200 before my next vacation starting April 1st. Last week, I was at 202. The weight loss pace has slowed down, which is understandable as there's not much left to lose. Initially, I was shedding around 12.5 pounds on average for four months straight, but now it's closer to 8 pounds a month.

As I look back on this journey, I find it both challenging and rewarding. I plan to take most of April as a break, especially with Easter around the corner and its tempting sweets.

To give you an idea of what I've been eating:

- Bacon and eggs with cheese (1 carb)

- NY Strip Steak with broccoli (2 carbs)

- Butter Garlic Chicken or steak with broccoli (2 carbs)

- Air-fried chicken wings with Wingstop Louisiana dry rub (2ish carbs for 9-10 wings)

- Cheeseburger with Costco Keto Hamburger buns and sugar-free ketchup (around 400 calories, 3 carbs)

- Tacos with Mama Lupes 0 carb tortillas (230ish calories per taco, 2 carbs with diced tomatoes, 1 carb without tomatoes)

- Steak or chicken Quesadillas with Mama Lupes 0 carb tortillas (170 calories, 0 carbs)

- 2x Tuna Sandwiches with Costco Keto bread (310 calories, 0 carbs)

- Brats with Walmart keto buns (150 calories per 3 carbs)

For snacks, I enjoyed:

- 28x Blue Diamond Smokehouse Almonds (170 calories, 2 carbs)

- Sweet cravings were satisfied with:

- 4x Soft Keto Friendly Aldi Cookies (130 calories, 2 carbs)

- Ratio Vanilla Keto Yogurt (200 calories, 2 carbs)

- Sugar-free jello (10 calories, 0 carbs)

- Quest frosted birthday cake cookies (90 calories, 1 carb)

- Sugar-free gum

This journey has been transformative, and I hope my story inspires others to embark on their path toward better health and financial well-being.

Running to Beat Diabetes

A week from today marks the third anniversary of my recommitment to running, and I'm thrilled to share my incredible journey. Over these three years, I've not only covered 4,136 miles but also transformed my life in more ways than one.

In my late 20s and early 30s, I was a dedicated runner, completing several half marathons and consistently logging 500-600 miles each year. However, life's demands and a few injuries gradually led to a decline in my running routine. By 2016, at the age of 37, I had only managed 288 miles for the year, with an average pace of 12:02, and my weight had ballooned from just over 200 pounds to just over 300.

My journey took an unexpected turn at the end of 2016 when I decided to reignite my fitness journey. However, an abrupt increase in miles resulted in severe back pain that prompted a doctor's visit. During this checkup, a routine examination revealed sugar and blood in my urine. This discovery set in motion a series of events that changed my life forever.

On Super Bowl Sunday in 2017, while the Atlanta Falcons were enduring a heartbreaking loss, I found myself running the highest fever I'd ever experienced. Believing it was the flu, I headed home after the game. However, my condition rapidly deteriorated, with uncontrollable shivering and intense cramping. A friend rushed me to the ER, where I was diagnosed with sepsis stemming from the bladder procedure I'd undergone earlier.

The hospital stay that followed was a life-altering experience. While receiving treatment for sepsis, I received another shocking diagnosis: Type 2 Diabetes, with an A1C of 9.1, indicating poor blood sugar control. It was a devastating blow.

Returning home, I was overwhelmed and defeated, weighing in at 303 pounds. My daily routine involved sitting on the couch for 45 minutes while I received my IV antibiotics, during which I decided to watch "Iron Man." Tony Stark's journey from captivity to building his first suit "in a cave, with a bunch of scraps" resonated with me.

Although I knew I couldn't become Iron Man, I realized I could choose not to be defeated by my diagnosis and health challenges. I resolved to combat diabetes through a better diet and running.

Initially, I couldn't run due to the pic line in my arm, so I focused on my diet, reducing carbs and incorporating healthier options like grilled chicken. As I recuperated from sepsis, my weight began to drop, and by the time I was cleared to run, I had already shed 18 pounds, reaching 285.

My first run post-recovery was on February 24th, 2017, covering 4 miles. It was more of a walk, but it marked the beginning of my comeback. The next day, I continued with 5 miles at a 13-minute pace.

Over the months that followed, I made significant progress. By March 2017, I had run 96 miles, and by the end of the month, I achieved a 4-mile run in under 40 minutes. The following month, I broke 100 miles, and by May, I completed my first 5K without walking and clocked in under 30 minutes.

This was just the start of my journey. By July, I was running 7 miles daily at a pace consistently below 10 minutes per mile. By December, I had reached 230 pounds and ran my first half-marathon in eight years, completing it in 1:54.

I've faced obstacles and setbacks along the way, from Achilles and patella tendinitis to a broken elbow. Nevertheless, I persevered, becoming faster, stronger, and healthier. A few months ago, I finally broke through the 230-pound barrier, and today, I weigh 208.

At my last check-up, my A1C had dropped to 5.7, returning to the non-diabetic range (though I'll continue managing it). My average pace for the 260 miles I've run this year is 8:53, including a remarkable 1:47:39 half marathon, almost 7 minutes faster than my previous attempt two years ago.

In these three years, I've run over four thousand miles, participated in numerous races, explored iconic locations like the Millennium Bridge in London and the Central Park 10K loop, and lost a staggering 95 pounds. At 40, I'm healthier than I was in my 30s, and I keep defying my own expectations.

My journey wasn't easy, but I never stopped lacing up my shoes and pushing myself down the road. That's the beauty of running – we're only competing with ourselves, and as long as we keep moving forward, we're winning.

My 28th Diabetes anniversary is next week

In the late November of 1990, when I was just six years old, my life took an unexpected turn when I was diagnosed with diabetes. Prior to my diagnosis, I had been feeling unwell for a couple of weeks, experiencing nausea, fatigue, and persistent headaches. My parents, initially believing it was a stomach bug, had been treating my symptoms with the usual homemade remedies, such as flavored ice and ginger ale (Vernors, for my fellow Michiganders).

However, a visit to the pediatrician changed everything. The doctor's first action was to check my blood sugar, and the result was alarming - it was over 700. This prompted an immediate hospitalization, where I spent the next four weeks. During my stay, I relied on an IV drip for nourishment and treatment. I affectionately named my IV stand "Fred." I must admit, I wasn't the easiest patient to handle, and it often took four nurses to change my IV or draw blood – one for each limb. This experience may have contributed to my lifelong aversion to needles.

Finally, on Christmas Eve of 1990, I was discharged from the hospital, still just a six-year-old child. Unfortunately, my young age meant that I was released to my parents without learning how to administer my own insulin injections. My mom, a dental assistant, took on the responsibility of administering my insulin until I reached an age where I could do it myself. This dependency on others for injections would become a recurring challenge in my life as a person with diabetes.

My childhood endocrinologist, though well-meaning, was somewhat lacking in his approach. Regardless of what I ate, the prescription remained the same: three units of insulin - two long-acting and one regular. He rarely monitored my A1C, perhaps checking it only once every 18 months. However, what he did have was a Super Nintendo with a game called Captain Novolin, which I found pretty awesome.

My first and only severe hypoglycemic episode occurred on Christmas Day in 1996 when I was 12 years old. Our family had a tradition of enjoying chocolate chip pancakes on Christmas morning. On that fateful day, after opening presents, my mom administered my insulin (as I still couldn't do it myself), and my dad was preparing to make the pancakes. However, I was given a dartboard and was eager to play. My dad and I went to my room to play darts, and that's when I lost consciousness.

I woke up to the sight of paramedics surrounding me. My blood sugar had plummeted to 22. The entire day was marred by a terrible feeling, and I knew that I had to make significant changes to better manage my diabetes.

In April 1997, at the age of 12, I received my first insulin pump, a manual infusion-only Distronic. Regrettably, I still couldn't manage the injections myself. My insulin regimen now consisted of Novolin, albeit only three units, primarily for meals like spaghetti or salad.

Fast forward to May 2007, I got married and bought a house. I was holding down a full-time job, but there was a catch - my (now ex) wife had to change my infusion sites. Over the following eight years, I pushed the limits of my infusion changes further and further. At one point, I was stretching them to the max, changing them every five weeks.

On December 26, 2015, I filed for divorce after discovering my ex-wife's infidelity. But focusing on my diabetic journey, marked the point where I had to learn to do my own infusions. You'd think it would be easy, especially with my Medtronic Paradigm Revel pump that featured a Quick-serter. All I had to do was push two buttons, yet it took me four hours on January 18, 2016, to summon the courage to do it for the first time in my life. I was 31 years old.

Over the next two years, I improved, and I could change my pump site in as little as 20 minutes. Still, it wasn't a breeze, and I was averaging a month between site changes.

In September 2017, I tied the knot for the second time. I showed my new wife how to change my site, and she did it twice, just in case I was ever unable to do it myself. However, I was adamant that it was my responsibility, not hers.

Then came the pivotal moment in August 2018 - I discovered I was going to be a father, initially expecting triplets, though we sadly lost one. Now, we were expecting twins, two boys. This was the catalyst for me to prioritize my health as a diabetic. I needed to be healthy and present to watch Alex and Ben grow up.

So, I started getting back on track with my infusion site changes, aiming to do them more consistently and on time. I even began exploring the possibility of obtaining a CGM through my insurance.

Diabetes is undeniably challenging, but it could be worse. Thankfully, there are medicines and technologies available to manage this condition, allowing me to live a life that's almost like anyone else's.

I just met the best gas station cashier

I found myself waiting in line at the gas station, purchasing some candy for my younger brother, when my insulin pump suddenly beeped, demanding my attention. My pump typically hung on my hip, making the tubing visible when I retrieved it from my pocket.

In the queue behind me stood a mother with her approximately nine-year-old child. I overheard the curious child's question and noticed they were gesturing toward my pump. Engrossed in dealing with the pump's alert, I initially disregarded their inquiry, my primary concern being my own health.

Unfortunately, my situation took an abrupt turn for the worse as my blood sugar began dropping too rapidly. Fumbling with my pump, I urgently needed to adjust my insulin dosing. Amidst this frantic process, I felt an unexpected, forceful push against my shoulder from behind.

Dizzy and off balance due to my plummeting blood sugar, I narrowly avoided a face plant thanks to the timely support of a nearby display countertop. Annoyed and bewildered, I turned around to find the child's mother glaring at me, her frustration palpable.

"Hey! Are you deaf or something? My kid asked you a question. What's that tube coming out of your stomach? You need to explain to my child what that is!" she demanded indignantly.

I couldn't help but wonder what had provoked this woman's outburst. I knew I owed no one an explanation about my insulin pump. Before I could formulate a response, the cashier interjected, sternly rebuking her for her inappropriate behavior. He promptly escorted her out of the store.

Despite the mother's protestations, she was unable to obtain the coveted Laffy Taffy for her child. In response to her disruptive behavior, the cashier even threatened to involve the police. The disgruntled mother eventually scurried away, like a chastised puppy.

After this tumultuous incident, the cashier kindly assisted me in picking up the items I had inadvertently dropped during the commotion. He also extended a sincere apology for the ordeal I had endured, inquiring about my well-being. To my surprise, he offered me a complimentary slice of freshly cooked pizza as a gesture of goodwill.

As I expressed my gratitude, I couldn't help but admire how the cashier had swiftly put the entitled mother in her place. It was, undoubtedly, a heartwarming display of justice being served.

I went into denial upon diagnosis

I thought I could bypass the process of dealing with this diagnosis, but as it turns out, I couldn't just sidestep the need to confront it head-on. It all started in late March when I decided to request another A1C test during a routine doctor's visit. Given my family history, I was aware of the risks and had been trying to stay vigilant, even though it had been two years since my last (and negative) test.

The results were alarming – my A1C was at ten, and my blood sugar had spiked to 400. The reality of it all hit me like a ton of bricks. Diabetes had cast a long shadow over my family, and my mother, out of concern, had once warned me, when I was about sixteen and had consumed two Jones sodas, that I might not live past the age of 35 due to diabetes. Sadly, I received my diagnosis just before my 35th birthday.

Initially, I chose to live in denial – perhaps it could be type 1 diabetes? (Even though I knew that type 1 isn't necessarily any easier to manage.) The blood tests, however, confirmed type 2. This made me realize that more people should routinely undergo these blood tests to catch such conditions early.

As time passed, I began to accept my diagnosis, driven by the desire to feel better day by day. I had come to understand that there was a stark difference in how I felt with blood sugar levels at 278 compared to 124. It was clear to me that my mother had expressed a genuine and valid fear but had conveyed it in a misguided way. We now know that if a mother has gestational diabetes, the risk of the child developing diabetes increases significantly. The genetic link is powerful, and our family might have approached prevention differently with this knowledge, if only we hadn't been so conflicted about our relationship with food. In hindsight, we would have extended that same focus to my brother, who, despite not being overweight, also carries a significant risk – genetics tend to be indifferent to appearances.

Now, I'm in a much better place. Knowledge is power, and I've learned that exercise efficiently transports glucose from the blood to the muscles while also enhancing insulin sensitivity for up to 24 hours. So, I've made a commitment to incorporate physical activity into my daily routine, whether it's an exercise video or a brisk walk before work.

I've adopted the Plate method advocated by the American Diabetes Association, leaning towards wholesome foods like salmon, onions, and Greek yogurt. My local grocery store offers pre-chopped vegetable boxes, which have been a game-changer for me in making healthier choices.

My treatment regimen includes Trulicity, Metformin, and insulin. I've developed quite an appreciation for Metformin, especially because I'd dealt with gastroparesis issues for years prior to my diabetes diagnosis. Despite the gastrointestinal side effects that many dislike, I feel like Metformin ensures my intestines keep functioning smoothly.

The Dexcom G6 continuous glucose monitor has been a transformative addition to my diabetes management. Something about seeing real-time information has had a profound impact on my behavior. I've started drinking more water to help flush out any lingering glucose and have even made an effort to use my CPAP machine consistently to manage my sleep apnea, knowing that these two conditions can exacerbate each other.

Insulin has turned out to be far less intimidating than I'd initially thought. I don't understand why it carries the stigma it does for people with type 2 diabetes. My dietitian shared a study that suggests if insulin is introduced early enough for type 2 diabetes, the pancreas can regain its functionality.

Needles no longer scare me, and I've finally mastered the proper use of a glucometer. It works much better when I insert the strip, hear that beep, and then patiently wait for the second beep.

While I still have a long way to go in managing my diabetes effectively, I've moved past the denial stage and haven't noticed any significant organ damage so far (fingers crossed). My goal is to keep it that way.

Living with diabetes is far from easy, but pointing fingers and assigning blame is ultimately futile. My dietitian pointed out that she's never seen anyone develop diabetes solely from their

diet; there's almost always a genetic component involved.
Perhaps more frequent testing could have made a difference;
who knows? I wish I had recognized those intense sweet
cravings as the warning signs they were.

But here I am, embracing the reality. Diabetes is a widespread
chronic illness that millions upon millions of people learn to
live with every day, and I can too. It doesn't mean I have to give
up all the delicious foods out there; it's simply an opportunity
to reevaluate the foods I enjoy (like discovering my newfound
love for onions).

My life in India with T1D

I have vivid memories of the events leading to my diabetes diagnosis, which took place on September 25th, 1992. I was just 11 years old at the time, and in a matter of seconds, my life took an unexpected turn. My parents, Mom and Papa, rushed me to our family doctor, who advised immediate hospitalization.

I spent the next 15 days in the hospital, and during this time, I had to come to terms with some significant changes. One of the first things I learned was that I could no longer enjoy my favorite treat, Dairy Milk. It felt like there was nothing sweet left for me.

A new chapter in my life had begun. Initially, Papa administered my insulin injections, but it wasn't long before I could manage them myself. My family was incredibly supportive, encouraging me to ignore the ignorant comments of others. However, the real challenge for me came at school, where some classmates began to tease and bully me with hurtful remarks.

I learned to rise above the negativity and focus on my studies. I became the top student in mathematics at the school, effectively silencing my critics. Suddenly, those same classmates wanted to be friends with me. I chose to pursue the

Science stream and managed to secure decent marks in Class 12th, even though I couldn't clear any competitive exams.

(That was in 1998.)

Following my parents' advice, I enrolled in a B.Sc. program at Rajdhani College of Delhi University while simultaneously preparing for engineering exams. It was during this time that a significant incident occurred.

One day, I experienced a hypoglycemic episode and began eating a snack on the college stairs to raise my blood sugar when a teacher confronted me. He abruptly confiscated my snacks, admonishing me for eating in a restricted area. This led to an argument, eventually escalating to the point where I was taken to the college principal. The principal made a hasty decision without hearing my side of the story and issued a suspension order.

I reached out to my mom, who promptly rushed to my side. She single-handedly confronted the college principal, leading to the order being revoked. This experience changed me, and I decided to redouble my efforts to prepare for engineering entrance exams.

In the midst of it all, I experienced a severe episode of ketoacidosis in June 1999, which was a harrowing ordeal. Fortunately, I was able to recover.

In July 1999, the results started rolling in, and although I didn't clear the Delhi College of Engineering exam, I secured admission to an engineering college in Moga, Punjab. This was a challenge because the insulin I needed was unavailable in Moga. Nevertheless, my parents managed to get me enrolled, and we sourced insulin from Ludhiana.

For the first time in my life, I found myself on my own, without any friends. I started a new life in Moga, where only a handful of people understood why I needed insulin. The rest assumed I was using drugs, but I took it all in stride.

One day, my father informed me about a new university opening in Delhi called Indraprastha University (GGSIPU). He sent me the application forms, and I managed to pass the entrance exams. Within three months, I was back home, a tremendous relief for me. I secured admission to Maharaja Agrasen Institute of Technology in Delhi in November 1999.

It was during college that I began my part-time business of assembling computers in my second year, even though my field of study was mechanical engineering. College life was enjoyable, and I made lasting friendships. In 2003, I graduated as an engineer, and I initially intended to prepare for the CAT exam, but life had different plans for me.

While preparing for the CAT exam, I met Richa online. We discovered that we both were preparing for the same exam and shared common interests. Eventually, I revealed to her that I was a diabetic and would need insulin for life. I also confessed my love for her, and to my delight, she reciprocated. We became a couple.

I decided to take over my Papa's business, which he had been running part-time until 2004. Though he was always there as a guiding force, I took on the responsibility of running the business, and it worked out well.

I introduced Richa to my parents, and they were thrilled about our relationship. Her parents were formally invited, and after much deliberation, we got married in January 2007.

We were blessed with two sons, with Amber being the elder one and Aarush the younger. However, in December 2016, our lives took an unexpected turn when our younger son, Aarush, was also diagnosed with Type 1 Diabetes. I was devastated and started blaming myself, but with the unwavering support of my wife and family, we made Aarush our top priority and ensured he received the care he needed.

On January 10, 2017, I made the decision to close my factory, and on February 6, 2017, I began a new chapter in my life by taking on the role of Senior Manager of Sales. As I write this today, it has been two months since I resigned from that job, and things are gradually improving.

Life is an everyday struggle, and we must confront and embrace the challenges it presents.

T1D since I was 14 years old

Type 1 diabetes (T1D) became a part of my life when I was just 14 years old, and surprisingly, it's one of the best things that ever happened to me.

Now, don't get me wrong – there's not much inherently "fun" about dealing with this condition, although I managed to turn it into a sort of badge of honor that made me somewhat popular in school.

What makes T1D a blessing is the invaluable life lessons it imparts. At the time of my diagnosis, I was given a stark revelation: if I had delayed seeing a doctor by just one more week—merely seven days—I could have ended up in a coma, or worse. This close brush with potential death at such a young age drastically altered my outlook on life. It hammered home the brevity of our time here and the uncertainty of how close we might be to the end. It taught me the importance of living life to the fullest.

Since that pivotal moment, I've evolved into a different person altogether. T1D has instilled in me a work ethic that I likely wouldn't have developed without it. It's motivated me to contribute positively to the world. This condition has nurtured empathy and discipline within me, with the simple act of choosing to pass on a tempting cookie becoming a formidable test of self-control. It has unveiled facets of my character that can only emerge from adversity.

Today, I stand as a stronger, healthier, and happier individual thanks to T1D.

Of course, it hasn't been all smooth sailing. I grappled with less-than-ideal blood sugar levels for years. It was only in the last three years that I finally uncovered a system that works for me. My A1C levels have plummeted from 8.0% and above to a much-improved range of 6.2% to 6.5%. Surprisingly, I now incorporate more carbs into my diet, and I savor the occasional chocolate and cookies, all within reasonable limits.

T1D isn't a sentence to imprisonment; it's more of a guiding presence in my life. It's a reminder that encourages me to scrutinize my habits and diet more meticulously than the average person. I don't view diabetes as my enemy; rather, it's been my ally from day one. Just like any friends or partners, we may occasionally want to throttle each other, but at the core, there's a deep mutual affection.

For me, T1D is the very essence of what defines me as a person.

Miraculous Postpartum: Escaping Preeclampsia's Grasp

Just four days after what seemed like a nearly perfect vaginal delivery, I found myself facing a life-threatening situation due to preeclampsia. My journey through pregnancy had been marked by various complications, but this unexpected turn of events taught me some crucial lessons about life and the importance of paying attention to one's health.

I should mention that my pregnancy was already considered high-risk. I had been diagnosed with gestational diabetes, which I managed with metformin. My weight was a concern, and I carried a family history of high blood pressure and diabetes. Alongside all of this, I grappled with bipolar disorder, which I managed effectively with a combination of medications throughout my pregnancy.

Despite these challenges, preeclampsia, a condition characterized by high blood pressure and often occurring during pregnancy, can affect anyone due to the profound hormonal changes involved.

Considering the complications, I had faced throughout my pregnancy, I had prepared myself for a challenging labor and delivery experience. I had even contemplated the possibility of a C-section due to concerns about having a larger baby. However, fate had other plans, and I ended up having a near-perfect delivery with a dedicated birthing team by my side. There was no vaginal tearing, and we welcomed a healthy baby boy with a full head of hair. Everything seemed to be going well, and we were discharged from the hospital just two days later.

However, the very next day, I began experiencing breathlessness and chest pressure. I attributed these symptoms to the normal postpartum recovery process, especially since I had been forewarned about the discomfort associated with the uterus returning to its normal size and organs shifting back into place. I continued with my daily routine, caring for the baby, organizing, and cleaning, but I took breaks to catch my breath.

As the day wore on, I started to notice heart palpitations. Although I initially brushed them off as anxiety, I couldn't ignore the persistent chest pressure and shortness of breath. It was only then that I remembered the potential risks of my high-risk pregnancy, and it dawned on me that I should check my blood pressure. Regrettably, I didn't do it right away because I felt I had too much to handle.

Eventually, I decided to take action, and my husband and I checked my blood pressure using a monitor we had at home. The reading was alarming—177/106, with a pulse of 66. I repeated the test several times, unable to believe the dangerously high readings. I naively thought that as long as it wasn't above 200, it should be okay.

My husband and I rushed to the emergency room, where the medical staff responded swiftly and with an air of urgency. Despite their efforts to keep the mood light, their speed made it evident that this was a serious situation. My blood pressure had spiked into the critical danger zone—190s/100s with a heart rate in the 60s.

The medical team faced challenges in starting an IV due to my thin veins, but they remained composed and light-hearted throughout. I engaged in conversation with them, grateful for their jokes and attempts to keep my spirits up. Little did I know that a blood pressure reading in the 190s was life-threatening, with the potential for strokes, seizures, or even a heart attack. Their prompt and calm actions were aimed at preventing such catastrophic events, and I was incredibly fortunate to be in a hospital that could handle the situation efficiently (Huntington Hospital in Pasadena, CA).

I was quickly hooked up to IVs, monitors, and leg compression wraps to prevent blood clots. I received a magnesium drip and a BP medication drip to stabilize my condition. While I wasn't out of the woods yet, my blood pressure had dropped from the danger zone. I would likely be discharged with BP medication after two days, but the experience had left me deeply shaken.

I couldn't help but reflect on how close I had come to losing my life. My baby could have been left without a mother, and my husband, who loves me deeply, would have been devastated. My mother, a retired nurse of 40 years, would have been unable to save me. I might have become a supporting character in a tragic story, and my son would never have had the chance to know his mother.

This experience has rattled me to my core, and I now carry a deep sense of gratitude for the second chance at life I've been given. My message to everyone is to take pregnancy complications seriously and ensure regular check-ups, including monitoring blood glucose levels and blood pressure. Gestational diabetes and preeclampsia can affect anyone, regardless of their circumstances. Hormones are indeed a force to be reckoned with, and we should always prioritize our health and well-being.

Inspirational Quotes

"I have high blood sugars, and Type 2 diabetes is not going to kill me. But I just have to eat right, and exercise, and lose weight, and watch what I eat, and I will be fine for the rest of my life."

Tom Hanks

"Diabetes just boggles me. I know when you get heart pain; I've had them. I don't know what diabetes feels like. ... If someone had said to me, 'What's your No. 1 health problem?' I would have said heart disease and then diabetes. And what doctors tell me now is that I can transpose them and say diabetes."

Larry King

"Diabetes sounds like you're going to die when you hear it. I was immediately frightened. But once I got a better idea of what it was and that it was something I could manage myself, I was comforted."

Nick Jonas

"Everyone has a challenge in life. There's always something you're overcoming…We get knocked down, but we can get back up. Chase your dreams. Rely on your support team. Find out what resources you have and use them. Don't let diabetes stop you."

Will Cross

"Don't let yourself fall, you gotta pick yourself right up and strive to do better and be better! Think positive. Don't let Diabetes control you! You control the Diabetes! Be strong because some ways might be tough but you are tougher!"

Tiffany Danczak

"When it comes to eating right and exercising, there is no 'I'll start tomorrow.' Tomorrow is a disease."

Terri Guillemets

"My diabetes is such a central part of my life… It did teach me discipline… it also taught me about moderation… I've trained myself to be super-vigilant… because I feel better when I am in control."

Sonia Sotomayor

"People take ownership of sickness and disease by saying things like MY high blood pressure MY diabetes, MY heart disease, MY depression, MY! MY! MY! Don't own it because it doesn't belong to you!"

Stella Payton

As you reach the end of '*Diabetic Chronicles: Life Stories of Diabetes Warriors,*' we hope these remarkable narratives have left a lasting impact on your heart and soul.

The strength, courage, and resilience displayed by these diabetes warriors serve as a testament to the indomitable spirit of the human journey. We invite you to carry their stories with you as a source of inspiration and hope in your own life.

Thank you for joining us on this inspiring journey. We encourage you to share these stories, connect with others, and continue the conversation about diabetes awareness and support.

With gratitude,

Tahar Das

Made with love